Father,

Thank you for the abilitie:
and wisdom we gain from

*Be with us as we work that we may do our best. Help us
to be encouraging to others in our daily life. Thank you
for the people that you have brought into our lives.*

*Bless the athletes, coaches, workout partners and all
those who support our training.
May the results from our training be a reflection of
Your Spirit in our lives.*

*Finally Father, remind us that there is no failure, but
only growth in the body, mind and Spirit.*

Amen

Contents

Copyright

Killer Kettlebell WOD Bible: 200+ Cross Training KB Workouts

First Edition – April 2014.

Written by P Selter

A Shredded-Society Publication
www.Shredded-Society.com

Disclaimer

The information provided in this book is designed to provide helpful information on the subjects discussed. This book is not meant to be used, nor should it be used, to diagnose or treat any medical condition. For diagnosis or treatment of any medical problem, consult your own physician. The publisher and author are not responsible for any specific health or allergy needs that may require medical supervision and are not liable for any damages or negative consequences from any treatment, action, application or preparation, to any person reading or following the information in this book. References are provided for informational purposes only and do not constitute endorsement of any websites or other sources. Readers should be aware that the websites listed in this book may change.

I recommend consulting a doctor to assess and/or identify any health related issues prior to making any dramatic changes to your diet or exercise regime.

Bonus Content

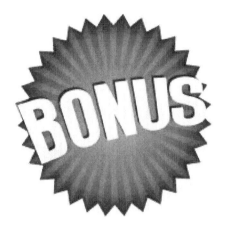

As a token of our appreciation Shredded-Society would like to give you access to our Cross Training exclusive bonus content.

<u>You're only a click away from receiving:</u>

The 5 most effective Cross Training workouts

A guide detailing the only Cross Training equipment you should use while training

Exclusive pre-release access to our latest eBooks

Free Shredded Society eBooks during promotional periods

Simply click here to receive this bonus content from Shredded-Society

As this is a limited time offer it would be a shame to miss out, I recommend grabbing these bonuses before reading on.

Introduction

I would like to thank you and congratulate you for purchasing the book, *Killer Kettlebell WOD Bible: 200+ Cross Training KB Workouts.*

This book will introduce you to the many health & fitness benefits of the phenomenon kettlebell training along with how to correctly perform common kettlebell exercises.

You will then be able to practise and implement these exercise with the 205 kettlebell WODs (workouts) contained within this book to improve your speed, strength and agility.

Thanks again for purchasing this book, I hope you enjoy it!

Benefits of Cross Training

Cross Training is not just a new fad amongst all the other styles of training that come and go throughout the years; Cross Training has many benefits these include:

Intensity

Cross Training workouts are fast paced and intense (as the emphasis is on speed and total weight being lifted), they are generally much shorter than a regular weight lifting workout – however since the workout is condensed it is constant non-stop movement, there is no time to stop and talk to your gym partner between sets like you normally would as you are constantly working against the clock to better yourself.

Creates Athletes

Cross Training exercises are all high power functional movements, this is highly emphasised. Cross Training, unlike bodybuilding does not believe in low power isolation movements. The major benefit here is now that the focus has been taken off vanity and looks it has been put 100% on performance – the core strength, stamina, coordination, agility and balance you will develop through participation in Cross Training will transfer over to sports and all other facets of life.

Time

The number one excuse for individuals not following a workout regime is the constraint of time; yes its true – working out takes time.

However, Cross Training WODs are short - with many intense workouts ranging from 15 – 20 minutes they are faster and more effective than a regular workout in which you spend an hour on a cross trainer mindlessly staring at the wall.

Measureable Results

Cross Training workouts provide you with measureable and repeatable data; this can be used to verify that your fitness level is increasing. With a series of 'bench mark' workouts known as 'The Girls' and 'The Heroes' you can easily assess your progress.

Life Changing

Change your body, change your life, and change your world…

Cross Training workouts build mental strength, grit and confidence; a tough Cross Training workout will emotionally push you beyond your limits. When you ignore the voice inside your head that says 'it's too hard' or 'I can't do that last rep' and push past it unbreakable confidence is built – then anything is possible.

Community

Cross Training encourages community, both in the gym and online.

People encourage and support each other through out their workouts – you will never have to work out alone again unless you want to, as the bond formed between training partners make training truly fun. It is very rarely you will find an individual that is as passionate about a particular pastime as yourself however this could not be further from the truth with the Cross Training community; we are all teammates that push and pray for each other.

Terminology

The following Cross Training terminology guide will come in helpful when interpreting your Cross Training workouts.

1RM: Your 1RM is your max lift for one rep

AHAP: as heavy as possible

AMRAP: As many rounds as possible

ATG: Ass to Grass

BP: Bench press

Box: Another name for a gym

BS: Back squat

BW: Body weight

CTT: Cross Training Total - consisting of max squat, press, and deadlift

CTWU: Cross Training Warm-up

Chipper: A WOD containing many different exercises and reps

CLN: Clean

C&J: Clean and jerk

C2: Concept II rowing machine

DL: Deadlift

DOMS: Delayed onset muscle soreness

DU: Double under

EMOM: Every minute on the minute

For Time: Timed workout, perform as quickly as possible and record score.

FS: Front squat

GHR(D): Glute ham raise (developer). Posterior chain exercise, similar to a back extension. Also, the device that allows for the proper performance of a Glute Ham Raise.

GHR(D) Situp: Situp performed on the GHR(D) bench.

GPP: General physical preparedness, another word for fitness

GTG: Grease the Groove, a protocol of doing many sub-maximal sets of an exercise throughout the day

H2H: Hand to hand; refers to Jeff Martone's kettlebell "juggling" techniques

HSPU: Hand stand push up. Kick up into a handstand (use wall for balance, if needed) bend arms until nose touches floor and push back up.

HSQ: Hang squat (clean or snatch). Start with bar "at the hang," about knee height. Initiate pull. As the bar rises drop into a full squat and catch the bar in the racked position. From there, rise to a standing position

IF: Intermittent Fasting

KB: Kettlebell

KBS: Kettlebell swing

KTE: Knees to elbows.

MetCon: Metabolic Conditioning workout

MP: Military press

MU: Muscle ups. Hanging from rings you do a combination pull-up and dip so you end in an upright support.

OH: Overhead

OHS: Overhead squat. Full-depth squat performed while arms are locked out in a wide grip press position above (and usually behind) the head.

PC: Power clean

Pd: Pood, weight measure for kettlebells

PR: Personal record

PP: Push press

PSN: Power snatch

PU: Pull-ups or push ups depending on the context in WOD

Rep: Repetition. One performance of an exercise.

RM: Repetition maximum.

ROM: Range of motion.

Rx'd: As prescribed, without any adjustments.

SDHP: Sumo deadlift high pull

Set: A number of repetitions. e.g., 34sets of 8 reps, often seen as 4x8, means you do 8 reps, rest, repeat, rest, repeat, rest, repeat.

SPP: Specific physical preparedness, aka skill training.

SN: Snatch

SQ: Squat

SS: Starting Strength; Mark Rippetoe's great book on strength training basics

Subbed: Substituted

T2B: Toes to bar. Hang from bar. Bending only at waist raise your toes to touch the bar, slowly lower them and repeat.

Tabata: A form of interval training comprised of 20 seconds on, 10 seconds off repeated for 8 rounds.

TGU: Turkish get-up

The Girls: A series of benchmark workouts named after girls

The Heroes: Brutal benchmark workouts in honour of fallen soldiers

TnG: Touch and go, no pausing between reps

WO: Workout

WOD: Workout of the day

YBF: You'll Be Fine

What is a Kettlebell

A kettlebell is a weight, primarily made out of cast iron, the physical appearance of a kettlebell resembles that of a cannonball with a looped handle. Kettlebells are used for performing cross training and ballistic style exercises which work on your cardiovascular endurance, strength and flexibility. Kettlebells range in weight from 5lbs to well over 100lbs.

Kettlebells were originally developed in Russia in the 1700s. in 1704 'Girya', Russian for 'kettlebell' was published in the Russian dictionary. During this time farmers used kettlebells to weigh their crops, grains and other goods. After farmers discovered they were also useful for displaying strength the Soviet Army adopted kettlebells for use in their physical conditioning programs and training in the 20th century. Kettlebells found their way to the United States in the early 1960s, in 2001 Pavel Tsatsouline developed the first Kettlebell instructor certification program.

Kettlebells were declared the 'Hot Weight of the Year' in 2002 by Rolling Stone, kettlebells are finally getting the exposure they deserve as individuals begin to see fantastic results from their training.

The kettlebells centre of mass is extended beyond the hand, unlike that of a dumbbell, this encourages ballistic swinging movements and provides an unstable force when handled.

As you'll soon find out kettlebell training has a plethora of benefits, there's literally hundreds of different exercise variations you can perform with a kettlebell or two!

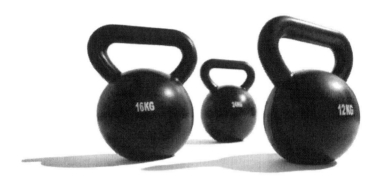

Benefits of Kettlebell Training

Cardio Becomes Fun

If you're looking to burn fat you no longer have to spend countless hours on the boring old treadmill. As stated earlier, kettlebell training incorporates modules of cardio along with functional strength and flexibility. Kettlebell workouts are short and intense; they will have you gasping for air and burning fat in fun, efficient manner unlike conventional steady state cardio.

Gain Functional Strength

The majority of exercises you will be performing with kettlebells are compound exercises, meaning they involve recruiting multiple muscle groups at once. By performing compound exercises such as the goblet squat, deadlift, clean and press and floor press with kettlebells your functional strength will greatly increase.

Improve Flexibility

Kettlebell exercises emphasize the postural muscles in a functional manner, resulting in increased flexibility and better posture.

Portable

Kettlebells, unlike barbells and the majority of other exercise equipment are portable. Now there's no excuse to miss a workout. Quite often when I go on holidays or are out of town for several days on business I take a couple of kettlebells with me, it's easy enough to do your kettlebell workout in large room or a public park.

Kettlebells Provide a Full Body Workout

Kettlebells provide you with a full body workout, swings, squats, snatches, deadlifts, lunges and presses are all compound exercises, working multiple muscle groups. The posterior chain is constantly being utilised during a kettlebell workout as the core must remain tight to assist in stabilising the swinging and rapid movement of weight.

Shock the System

Chances are if you're reading this you may not have trained with kettlebells before, and that's fantastic! If you're used to exercises with machines or dumbbells and hit a plateau (you are unable to gain size or progress to heavier weights) then switching to a kettlebell based workout regime for a period of time will shock the body into new growth, not to mention it's fun and a change of scenery – great for breaking the monotony of the gym.

Save Money

Kettlebells are cheap, generally in the $2-3 per kilogram price bracket. $100 spent on kettlebells is money well spent! You will not find such value for money in a gym membership or overpriced exercise equipment that produces minimal results. To get in great shape and build functional fitness a pair or 2 of the correct weight kettlebells is all you will need.

Develop Core Strength

Kettlebells will have you engaging your core on almost every exercise. Your lower back and core will gain tremendous strength and stability from performing exercise such as kettlebell swings, snatches, standing overhead presses etc. that said it is imperative to ensure you are using correct form, and tightening the core as necessary, otherwise you are leaving yourself susceptible to a lower back injury.

Improve Coordination

Kettlebell training will increase your hand eye coordination, as you are swinging and passing the kettlebell around your brain and muscles must coordinate correctly in order to perform the movements necessary. This increase coordination will transfer across to all of your athletic endeavours.

Correct Imbalances

Everybody has imbalances within their body, as if you're used to training with machines or barbells you will typically find you have a stronger side, which will compensate for the weaker side when necessary (many individuals find this apparent on pressing movements such as the overhead press and bench press). Kettlebell training will swiftly identify and correct imbalances through single limb exercises.

Save Time

Kettlebell workouts are short and intense, the majority of kettlebell workouts within this book can easily be completed within 10 – 20 minutes, if you find your workouts are taking substantially longer it is time to decrease your rest periods and increase your intensity. Many individuals dismiss working out due to lack of time, however when you have a portable set of kettlebells, and only require 15 – 20 minutes for an intense workout there are no valid excuses.

Develop Explosive Power

Performing Olympic lifts such as the clean & jerk and snatch will increase your explosive power drastically, and places a new spin on these exercises as opposed to performing them with a barbell or dumbbells.

Common Kettlebell Exercises

The following pages detail the correct form (technique) including a photo displaying the starting and finishing for common kettlebell exercises found in the workouts section of this book.

If you are completely new to kettlebell training I highly recommend training with a partner or coach whom has experience with kettlebells as incorrect form can easily lead to back injuries due to the amount of stress placed on the posterior chain when performing kettlebell swings etc.

Kettlebell American Swing

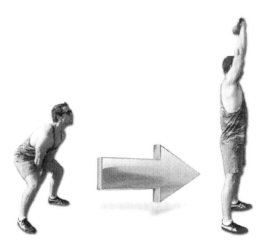

Note: Ensure you have mastered the Russian swing before progressing to the American swing.

Start with your foot positioning slightly wider than shoulder width, toes pointing straight forward.
The power for the American swing is all in your hips, ensure your back is straight, bend your knees and engage

your lats to pick up the weight and commence the swing. keep your arms slightly bent, stop the kettlebell swing overhead – you should not need to recruit your shoulders for the final part of the exercise, all power is to come through the hips, with engaged lats (many beginners drive through their front deltoids to get the kettlebell from chest height to overhead). The kettlebell should essentially float to the overhead position, with your lats being used to stop the weight at the top of the rep.

Kettlebell Russian Swing

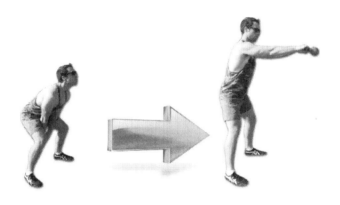

Start with your foot positioning slightly wider than
shoulder width, toes pointing straight forward.
The power for the Russian swing is all in your hips,
ensure your back is straight, bend your knees and engage
your lats to pick up the weight and commence the swing
keeping your arms slightly bent, stop the swing at chest
height by engaging the lats. ensure your core is tight for
the duration of your set.

Kettlebell Clean and Press

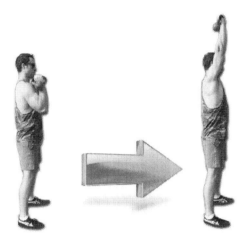

To begin push your glutes backwards and look straight ahead to ensure your back remains straight, extend through your hips and legs as you lift the kettlebells to shoulder height, rotating your wrists at the same time. Extend your elbow while rotating your palm forward to complete the press. Lower the kettlebell back to the starting position.

Kettlebell Row

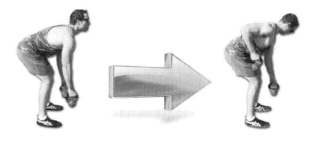

To begin push your glutes backwards and look straight ahead to ensure your back remains straight, hold onto both kettlebells by their handles. Retract your shoulder blade to draw one kettlebell towards your rib cage. Lower the kettlebell back to the starting positioning, proceed to row the second kettlebell by following the same protocol.

Kettlebell Goblet Squat

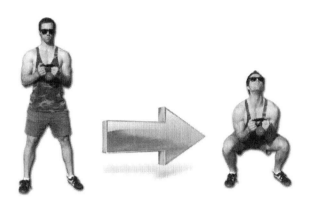

Grasp a kettlebell in front of your chest with both hands, ensure your elbows are tucked in as close to your body as possible. To begin the squat drive your hips backwards until your thighs are parallel to the floor. Return to an upright position by driving through your heels and keeping your core tight, look forward as you do so to ensure your back does not round.

Kettlebell Lunges

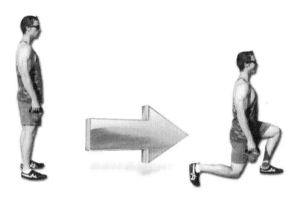

Hold 1 kettlebell in each hand by the handle, palms facing towards your body with your feet in a shoulder width stance. Step forward with one leg while flexing that knee to drop the hips, lower yourself until your rear knee brushes the ground. To complete the repetition flex both knees and drive through the heel of your front foot. Repeat with opposite leg, lunges can be performed either stationary or walking.

Kettlebell Russian Twists

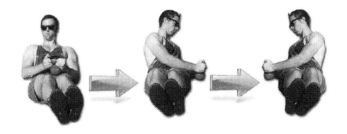

Sit on the ground, holding a kettlebell against your chest.
Lean back to a 45 degree angle, keep your legs straight,
slightly raised so they are not touching the floor.
Rotate your torso from side to side while holding the
kettlebell by twisting at the waist and moving the
kettlebell across your body, the further you lean back the
harder this exercise becomes.

Kettlebell Deadlifts

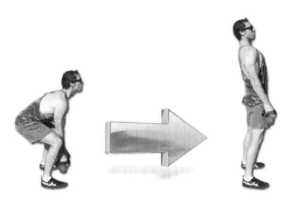

Begin with a kettlebell on the floor between your legs. Squat down to hold onto the kettlebell by dropping your hips and driving your glutes backwards while looking forward to ensure your back does not round. Hold the kettlebell with both hands, tighten your core and glutes before driving through your heels to lift the kettlebell until your arms are fully extended and shoulders are pushed back. Bend your knees as you slowly lower the kettlebell to the starting position to complete the rep.

Kettlebell Push Press

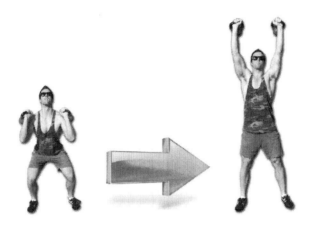

Proceed to clean a pair of kettlebells to shoulder height.
squat down several inches by dropping your hips and
driving your glutes backwards, use your explosive power
to now drive the kettlebells upwards, use the momentum
gathered to push the kettlebells overhead until locked
out.
Proceed to lower the kettlebells to the clean position
(shoulder height) to complete the rep.

Kettlebell Snatches

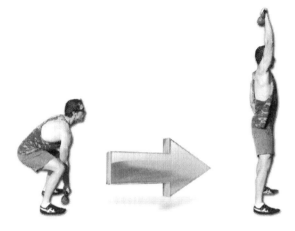

Begin with a kettlebell between your legs, drop your hips back and bend your knees to lower yourself to the starting position.

Grasp the kettlebell with one hand.

While looking forward swing the kettlebell backwards (between your legs) to gain momentum.

Swing the kettlebell forward while driving through your hips and knees; this will propel the kettlebell upwards.

Lock the weight out directly overhead by rotating your hand and punching straight up.

Proceed to lower the kettlebell down to the starting position.

Kettlebell Push-Ups

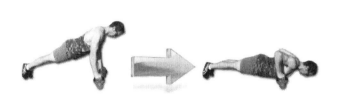

Begin with a pair of kettlebells on the ground at a slightly wider than shoulder width distance apart. Assume a pushup position by grasping the handle of each kettlebell.

Begin to lower your body until your arms are parallel to the floor, push back up – locking out your elbows to complete the repetition. The kettlebell pushup will allow a far greater range of motion than that of a regular pushup.

Kettlebell Thruster

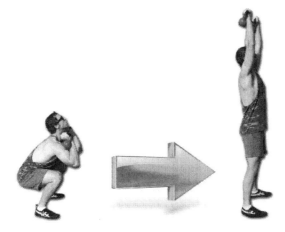

Begin by cleaning 2 kettlebells to shoulder height (clean by dropping your hips back as you push the kettlebells towards your shoulders).

Squat down by driving your hips backwards until your thighs are parallel to the floor. Return to an upright position by driving through your heels, while doing so extend your arms using the momentum of the squat to drive the kettlebells overhead.

Lower kettlebells to the starting position.

Kettlebell Floor Press

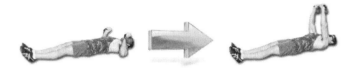

Lay on the floor with a kettlebell in each hand, your upper arm should be supported by the floor.

Proceed to press the kettlebell towards the roof by extending your elbows, as you press rotate your wrists until your palms are facing away from your face.

Lower the kettlebells until your upper arm touches the floor to complete the rep.

Kettlebell Turkish Get Up (TGU)

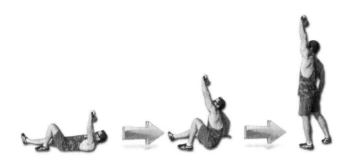

Note: I recommend practising the TGU without a kettlebell to ensure you have the movements correct before adding weight into the equatio

Lay on the floor with 1 kettlebell locked out overhead (in a one arm floor press position). Bend the knee of the side that is holding the kettlebell.

While ensuring the kettlebell remains in a locked out position for the duration of the exercise pivot your body to the opposite side of the kettlebell and use your free hand to drive forward into a lunge position before assuming a seated/squat like position.

While looking upwards at the kettlebell proceed to stand up.

Reverse the motion back to the floor while maintaining the locked out kettlebell to complete the repetition.

KB Farmers Walk

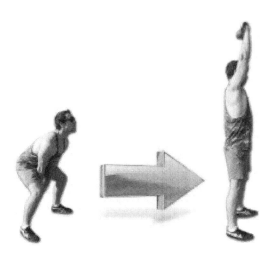

Stand in the middle of 2 kettlebells.
Firmly grip the handles of the kettlebells, proceed to lift them by driving through your heels, ensuring your back remains straight by keeping your head up.
Walk forward taking short, quick steps. Focus on your breathing as you move for the described distance.

Common Kettlebell Training Mistakes

Disregarding exercise progression:
As a beginner to kettlebells it is imperative that the foundation kettlebell exercises such as the deadlift and Russian swing are mastered first before attempting more advanced exercises such as the American swing.

Your fitness journey is a marathon, not a sprint so ensure you are progressing at a slow but consistent rate, if necessary hire a trainer to develop you a progressive exercise plan.

Using the upper body to muscle the kettlebell up:
The ballistic movements incorporated within kettlebell training should not require any drastic intervention from the upper body. A good example of this is attempting to 'muscle up' the kettlebell to the overhead position when performing a snatch or American swing. The upper body should remain relaxed during these movements as the hips are snapped and knees are locked for correct flow of the kettlebell.

Training to failure:

When training with dumbbells or barbells it is quite common to train to failure during your sets, many people carry this technique over when training with kettlebells. Training to failure when using kettlebells is a recipe for disaster as your form begins to deteriorate on your final reps the quality of your swing and overhead pressing/catching of the kettlebell can lead to serious shoulder and lower back injuries. When training with kettlebells it is highly recommended to stop several reps short of failure.

Using a 'death grip':

When holding onto your kettlebells grasp the handles with the hooks of your fingers as opposed to your palm as you run the risk of hand and elbow injuries when gripping the kettlebell too tight during ballistic movements.

Injuring forearms:
When performing exercises in which the kettlebell changes position during the movement such as kettlebell cleans and snatches ensure you are staying in control of

the kettlebell as it rotates to avoid any forearm damage due to being out of control as the kettlebell smashes down onto your forearm.

The best way to avoid this is to punch the kettlebell upwards as opposed to swinging it while slightly relaxing your grip to catch it before it falls and hits your forearm.

Incorrect footwear:
Running shoes are for running, not kettlebell workouts. Running shoes tend to have a slightly raised heel which is known to push your knees forward during exercises such as squats and swings. This will expose you to the risk of a knee injury.
Training barefoot is ideal for your stability, however if this is not an option I recommend training in flat soled shoes such as Chuck Taylors.

Kettlebell WODs

On the following pages you will find 205 kettlebell based WODs.

The exercises these workouts contain are single and dual kettlebell based, if you do not have access to 2 kettlebells simply scale these to single arm and either double or divide the repetitions based on your ability.

Have fun with it! Challenge your friends to beat your time and rounds on these WODs, after all fitness is all about having fun!

KB WOD 1

2 rounds:

50x Kettlebell Hand-to-hand swings

25x Kettlebell Double bottoms-up press

12x Kettlebell Snatch

50x Push-ups

KB WOD 2

For time:

Run 1 mile

100x KB snatch

200x Alternating KB press

300x KB swing

Run 1 mile

KB WOD 3

18 rounds:

1-2-3-2-3-4-3-4-5-4-5-6-5-6-7-6-7-8x reps

Double clean

Jerk

KB WOD 4

For time:

40x Plyo push-ups using KB handles

40x Hanging guard sit-ups

40x Pull-ups

40x Bench press

40x KB swing

40x Alternating KB press

Row 50 calories

KB WOD 5

AMRAP in 10 minutes:

1x Double KB snatch

2x KB Sotts press

3x KB thrusters

4x Push-ups

KB WOD 6

For max rounds:

On-the-minute Double KB Sumo deadlift

Start at 1 rep, add another rep at top of each minute

Continue until you cannot perform the requisite number of reps per round

KB WOD 7

Max reps in 10 minutes

Switch arms as necessary, KB may not touch floor

Long cycle KB clean & jerk

KB WOD 8

1 round:

Row 2km

200x KB swings

Row 2000m

KB WOD 9

8 rounds:

8x Single arm KB thruster

8x Pistol squats

8x KB reverse lunge

KB WOD 10

13 rounds:

21-18-15-12-9-6-3-6-9-12-15-18-21x reps

KB swings

Push-ups

KB WOD 11

3 rounds - 21-15-9x reps:

KB sumo high-pull

Double KB push jerk

KB WOD 12

AMRAP in 12 minutes:

3x KB pistol squats

6x Double KB snatch

9x KB jerk

KB WOD 13

Max rounds:

On the minute every minute perform

1x KB snatch first minute, then rest

2x KB snatch second minute, then rest

3x KB snatch third minute...

Continue until failure

KB WOD 14

18 rounds:

1-2-3-2-3-4-3-4-5-4-5-6-5-6-7-6-7-8x reps

Double snatch

Thruster

KB WOD 15

Max rounds:

On-the-minute Double KB Snatch

Start at 1 rep, add another rep at top of each minute

Continue until you cannot perform the requisite number

of reps per round

KB WOD 16

For time:

Use single KB

25x Ring dips

25x Walking lunges w/ KB overhead

50x Hand-to-hand swing

25x Walking lunges w/ KB overhead

50x Pull-ups

25x Ring dips

KB WOD 17

Max rounds in 12 minutes:

7x KB snatch

7x Ball slams

7x GHD sit-ups

KB WOD 18

5 rounds:

KB swings 80-40-20-40-80x

Push-ups 40-20-10-20-40x

Pull-ups 20-10-5-10-20x

KB WOD 19

3 rounds:

21-15-9x reps

KB sumo high-pull

Double KB push jerk

KB WOD 20

Max rounds in 7 minutes:

3x Back squat (bw)

6x Double KB swing (1/2 bw)

9x Push-ups

KB WOD 21

5 rounds:

20x Hand to hand KB swing

10x Double KB clean

20x Alternating bent KB row

10x Thruster

KB WOD 22

3 rounds:

5x Double KB snatch

10x Thrusters

20x Renegade rows

KB WOD 23

5 rounds:

All exercises are double KB

6x Front squat

6x Clean

6x Press

15x Swing

6x Bent over row

10x Burpees

KB WOD 24

Max rounds in 20 minutes;

3x KB snatch, each arm

5x Burpees

KB WOD 25

10 rounds:

6x KB snatch, each arm

12x Box jumps

KB WOD 26

4 rounds:

10-20-30-40x reps

KB swing

Man-makers

Alternating floor press

KB WOD 27

For max distance:

KB Farmer's walk for 12 minutes

Stop at top of each minute and do 5x burpees

KB WOD 28
3 rounds:
21-15-9x reps
KB thrusters
Ring pull-ups

KB WOD 29
For time:
75x KB snatch

KB WOD 30
For time:
53x KB swing
53x KB sumo deadlift high-pull
53x KB snatch
53x KB back extension

KB WOD 31
Max rounds in 15 minutes;
10x KB suitcase deadlift
Farmer's walk - 20 steps

KB WOD 32
For time:
20x KB swing
30x Single KB thruster, left arm
20x Push-ups
30x Sit-ups
20x KB sumo deadlift high pull
30x Burpees

20x Double KB snatch
200m Farmer's walk
20x KB swing

KB WOD 33
29 rounds:
Breathing ladder
KB swing

KB WOD 34
3 rounds:
5x Burpees
10x KB thrusters
15x KB sumo deadlift high-pull
20x Sit-ups

KB WOD 35
For time:
Use single KB
25x Ring dips
25x Walking lunges w/ KB overhead (left arm)
50x Hand-to-hand swing
25x Walking lunges w/ KB overhead (right arm)
50x Pull-ups
25x Ring dips

KB WOD 36
Max rounds in 12 minutes:
3x Clean
3x Front squat

3x Double Snatch

3x Bent row

KB WOD 37

5 rounds:

21x Sumo deadlift high pull

21x Burpees

Row 250m

KB WOD 38

3 rounds:

5x Double KB sumo deadlift

10x KB Goblet squat

40m Overhead carry

25x KB swings

KB WOD 39

3 rounds:

6x KB turkish get-up

6x KB clean/press/windmill combo

50m Heavy sandbag carry

KB WOD 40

For time:

Use two KBs for all weighted movements.

12x KB swing

12x Snatch

12x Clean & jerk

12x Bent rows

12x Burpees

12x High pulls

12x Mountain climbers

12x Sotts press

12x Suitcase swings

12x Push-ups on KB handles

KB WOD 41

3 rounds:

15x KB swings

15x each arm KB clean & jerk

15x KB goblet squats

30 KB Hand-to-hand swings

15x each arm KB snatch

KB WOD 42

Max rounds in 15 minutes:

Use single KB for all movements, KB may not touch floor

1x Snatch

1x Overhead squat

1x Windmill

1x Jerk

1x Hand-to-hand swing

KB WOD 43

For time:

400m KB Farmer's walk

50x Bottoms-up single KB thruster
25x/arm KB snatch
50x Alternating floor press
400m KB Farmer's walk

KB WOD 44

3 rounds:
KB snatch intervals, count total reps for score
10:10
20:10
10:10
30:10
15:10
25:60

KB WOD 45

For time:
Use single KB
25x Ring dips
25x Walking lunges w/ KB overhead (left arm)
50x Hand-to-hand swing
25x Walking lunges w/ KB overhead (right arm)
50x Pull-ups
25x Ring dips

KB WOD 46

For time:

50x reps of the following KB complex:

1x Snatch + 1x Push-press + 1x Reverse TGU + 1x
Hand-to-hand swing

KB WOD 47

3 rounds:

Double unders 42-30-18x reps

KB swings 21-15-9x reps

KB WOD 48

10 rounds:

KB Snatch 10-9-8-7-6-5-4-3-2-1x

Burpee 1-2-3-4-5-6-7-8-9-10x

KB thruster 10-9-8-7-6-5-4-3-2-1x

KB WOD 49

5 rounds:

20x Hand to hand KB swing

10x Double KB clean

20x Alternating bent KB row

10x Thruster

KB WOD 50

3 rounds:

21-15-9x

Knees to elbows

KB Turkish get-ups

Sit-ups

KB swings

Ring push-ups

KB WOD 51

AMRAP in 12 minutes:

3x Clean

3x Front squat

3x Double Snatch

3x Bent row

KB WOD 52

1 round:

Keep KB off the ground for the entire workout

200x KB swings

150x KB snatch

100x 1-arm KB press

KB WOD 53

Utilise 2 KBs for the following workout:

10x Front squat

20x Alternating bent row

10x Push press
10x Snatch

KB WOD 54
9x KB suitcase deadlift
12x/arm KB snatch
15x KB push press

KB WOD 55
30x KB front squat
30x Push-ups
10x KB snatch
10x Pull-ups, strict

KB WOD 56
20-14-8.
Kettlebell swings.
KB Clean and Press (Place on floor and alternate arms each rep)
Turkish Get Up(alternate arms each rep)

KB WOD 57
4 rounds:
Circuit: 5 rounds of :30 work, minute rest between rounds
Clean, :30 per side
Slingshot, :30 each direction
Thruster, :30 right

2-hand swing, :30
Thruster, :30 left
Push ups, :30
Sit ups, :30

KB WOD 58

20 seconds work/10 seconds rest of the following:
Kettlebell swings
push ups
kettlebell high pulls
goblet squats
thrusters
one arm rows
jumping jacks
bicycles

KB WOD 59

20 seconds work/10 seconds rest of the following:
kettlebell snatch right
kettlebell snatch left
mountain climbers

KB WOD 60

20 seconds work/10 seconds rest of the following:
kettlebell high pull
kettlebell thruster
Jumping jacks or jump rope

KB WOD 61

20 seconds work/10 seconds rest of the following:

Slam Bells

Squat Thrust

Flutter Kicks

KB WOD 62

20 seconds work/10 seconds rest of the following:

kettlebell snatch right

kettlebell snatch left

mountain climbers

kettlebell high pull

kettlebell thruster

Jumping jacks or jump rope

Slam Bells

Squat Thrust

Flutter Kicks

KB WOD 63

1 clean + 1 press + 1 squat + 1 renegade row per arm

2 clean + 2 press + 2 squat + 2 renegade row per arm

3 clean + 3 press + 3 squat + 3 renegade row per arm

Repeat, increasing reps as many times as possible

KB WOD 64

4 Rounds of 3 mins of work, 1 min of rest:

3x kbell cleans

6x kbell sh to oh

9x air squat

KB WOD 65

3 rounds:

box jump 10,8,6

3x sandbag TGU's

3x sandbag kettlebell walk 35ft

20x KB hand-to-hand

KB WOD 66

5 rounds:

2 cleans

1 squat clean

1 thruster

6 walking lunges with bells in the rack

jerk to overhead walk back

KB WOD 67

8-7-6-5-4-3-2-1

fronts squats

clean & push press/jerk
lunge

KB WOD 68
4 rounds:
15 air squats
10 dual swing to high pull
5 hindu pushups

KB WOD 69
4 rounds:
2 cleans
1 squat clean
1 thruster
6 walking lunges with bells in the rack
jerk to overhead walk back

KB WOD 70
7 rounds:
3 push press
walk oh
3 windmills
walk oh
3 pushups

KB WOD 71
EMOM for 3 minutes:
3 power cleans
5 pushups

KB WOD 72
4 rounds:
8 dual swings with catch release
5 burpees
2 sandbag getups with a walk down and back

KB WOD 73
1 minute snatch, left, medium weight
1 minute rest
1 minute snatch, right, medium weight
1 minute rest
30 secs snatch, left, ahap
1 minute rest
30 secs snatch, right, ahap

KB WOD 74
4 sprawls with deadlifts (dual KB)
3 dual deadlifts
2 dual cleans

1 dual thruster

25 yard farmer's carry, one up one down, switch, walk back

every third round run 200m without KB

KB WOD 75

3 rounds:

5 dual kb front squats

50 meter band sprint

KB WOD 76

3 min Russian KB swings

1 min rest

2 min Russian KB swings

1 minute rest

1 min Russian KB swings

KB WOD 77

8-6-4-3-2-1

dual cleans

dual front squats

dual push jerks

KB WOD 78

2 rounds:

200m run

30 uppercuts

200m run

30 walking lunges

200m run

30 kb situps

200m run

Kb WOD 79

3 rounds:

15 KB snatch

12 in & outs

9 pushups

6 burpees

KB WOD 80

5 rounds:

12 push press, total, 6/6

2 shuttle runs

8 swing to lunge, total

KB WOD 81

3 rounds:
all left, all right
5 KB power cleans
4 KB thrusters
3 KB push press
2 overhead squat

KB WOD 82

4 rounds:
10 kb lunges with pass
5 wall walks
10 dual KB sumo deadlift

KB WOD 83

5 rounds:
10 dual KB swings
10 dual KB swings with release/catch
10 dual KB swings with a flip

KB WOD 84

3 rounds:
800m run

21 box jumps
dual alt press, 8l/8r
21 single bell situps

KB WOD 85
5 rounds:
8 dual bell alternating bent over row (4r/4l)
5 dual bell kb cleans
1 dual bell kb thruster

KB WOD 86
7 rounds:
3 dual bent over row
3 dual cleans
3 dual front squats
3 dual alt push press (6 total reps)
3 dual thrusters

KB WOD 87
3 rounds:
100m run
15 jumping air squats
12 dual snatches
9 dual push jerks

KB WOD 88

5 rounds:
3 dual swing to high pull
3 dual cleans
3 dual front squats

KB WOD 89
3 rounds:
3 minutes of snatches
snatch every 10 seconds, rest overhead
switch hands as often as you like

KB WOD 90
9-6-3
dual sumo deadlift
dual clean and jerk
dual floor press

KB WOD 91
7 minute amrap
1 pullup
1 burpee
1 KB swing
2, 2, 2
3, 3,3
1, 1, 1
2, 2, 2

KB WOD 92

5-4-3-2-1

front squats

find your 1 rep max – hold as many KBs as necessary

12 min cap

KB WOD 93

3 minutes of single arm jerks

2 minutes of pullups

1 minute of burpees

3 minutes of rest

3 minutes of single arm jerks

2 minutes of pullups

1 minute of burpees

KB WOD 94

4 rounds:

12 dual cleans

50 yard walk with bells in the rack

200m sprint

KB WOD 95

5 rounds:

6 alternating floor presses (dual bells, one up one down)

1 minute rest

KB WOD 96

2 rounds:

1 minute dual kb snatch

1 minute tabata burpees

1 minute dual kb jerk

1 minute tabata burpees

KB WOD 97

3 rounds:

20 kb squats

10 Russian KB swings

5 sa swings. l

5 sa swings, r

KB WOD 98

7-5-3

dual bent over row

dual power clean

dual push press

KB WOD 99

2 rounds:

21 push press

400m run

21 cleans

400m run

21 front squats

KB WOD 100

20 yard sprint

20 secs rest while walking back

20 yard sprint

20 secs rest while walking back

20 power swings immediately followed by

30 yard sprint

20 secs rest while walking back

30 yard sprint

20 secs rest while walking back

20 power swings immediately followed by

40 yard sprint

20 secs rest while walking back

20 power swings

KB WOD 101

2 rounds:

6 minutes tabata

dual Russian KB swings

dual KB swing to high pull

dual KB snatch

KB WOD 102

EMOTM

5 snatch left

5 snatch right

5 burpees

KB WOD 103

6 rounds:

7 dual clean and jerk

20 foot sled pull

5 pullups

KB WOD 104

3 rounds:

3 reps each of

squat clean

thruster

push press/jerk

oh squat

all left, all right

KB WOD 105

2 rounds:

KB power clean

KB front squat
KB thruster
KB snatch to backwards lunge
1 all left, 1 ll right
2 all left, 2 all right
3 all left, 3 all right

KB WOD 106

3 rounds:
12 power swings
4 burpees
200m run
12 powers
8 burpees
200m run
12 powers
12 burpees
200m run

KB WOD 107

3 rounds:
5 burpees
7 KB front squats
9 american KB swings

3 over-unders

KB WOD 108

10 minutes of:
1 strict press
2 push press
3 push jerk

KB WOD 109

6 rounds:
2 KB cleans
2 KB clean to front squat
2 KB clean to thruster
2 KB overhead lunges

KB WOD 110

4 rounds:
25 strict KB press
25 KB push press
25 KB push jerk

KB WOD 111

3 rounds:
25 goblet squat
25 overhead squat, left
25 overhead squat, right

KB WOD 112

5 rounds:

5 burpees on the minute every minute

50 Russian KB swings

25 KB snatches, total

25 KB thrusters, total

KB WOD 113

8 minutes amrap:

5 front squats

7 russians

9 pushups

KB WOD 114

9-7-5-3-1

kb lunge with pass

kb pushups

kb situps

KB WOD 115

5 rounds:

10 burpee pullups

10 dual kb alt strict press

10 dual russians

200m run

KB WOD 116

dual KB floor press

2 presses every 30 seconds for 5 minutes

total of 20 reps

KB WOD 117

3 rounds:

all exercises are dual KB

8 sumo dl

6 swing to high pull

4 snatch

KB WOD 118

3 rounds:

1 minute single bell clean and jerk, each arm

1 minute rest

3 rounds

move up in weight each round

KB WOD 119

1 round:

650m run

15 burpees

35 Russian KB swings

250m run

15 burpees

35 Russian KB swings

650m run

KB WOD 120

7 rounds:

3 box jumps

3 push ups

6 American KB swings

9 air squats

KB WOD 121

5 rounds:

5 dual kb sumo deadlift

1-2-3-4-5 pushups/wall walks

5 knee to elbow

KB WOD 122

13 rounds:

3 strict KB press

3 KB push press

3 KB push jerk

KB WOD 123

8 minute amrap

12 dual KB sumo deadlifts

6 plyometric pushups

KB WOD 124

1 minute max effort at each station

90 seconds of rest between stations

American KB swings

pushups

sandbag ground to overhead

toes to bar

KB WOD 125

5 rounds:

dual KB swing x1

dual KB clean x2

dual KB squat x3

KB WOD 126

2-4-6-8-10-12-14-12-10-8-6-4-2

Russian KB swings

KB situps

KB WOD 127

3 rounds:
20 dual KB squat cleans
15 pushups
10 pullups

KB WOD 128

7 rounds:
3 sumo dead lift

KB WOD 129

12-9-6
dual kb swings
pullups

KB WOD 130

6 rounds:
3 single arm swings
3 KB cleans
3 KB split jerk

KB WOD 131

2 rounds:

100ft walking lunge, no KB

100ft walk with KB overhead

25 single arm KB swings

KB WOD 132

2 rounds:

200m farmers walk (dual)

35 KB wall ball (single)

200m farmers walk (dual)

KB WOD 133

amrap in 15 minutes:

10 KB dual alternating floor press

10 power swings

10 lunge with pass

10 sit-up

KB WOD 134

2 rounds:

10 KB deadlift

10 single arm KB swings

10 KB push press

all left, followed by right

KB WOD 135
10-8-6-5-4-3-2-1
dual KB floor press
pullups
horn squat

KB WOD 136
3 rounds:
2 KB presses
4 KB jerks
6 KB thrusters

KB WOD 137
3 dual kb deadlifts
5 dual kb cleans
7 dual kb jerks
5 rounds

KB WOD 138
21-15-9
KB squat clean
pushups
single arm KB situp

KB WOD 139
3 rounds:
25 single arm swings, each arm

50 Russian KB swings

25 push press, each arm

KB WOD 140

2 rounds:

600m run

10 dual KB clean, press and squat

10 pushups

3 TGU's

KB WOD 141

10 minutes amrap

5 snatch to overhead squat to thruster

each side, complete all three movements without putting
the KB down

KB WOD 142

20 minutes amrap

14 dual KB alternating press

14 dual KB alternating clean

KB WOD 143

12 minutes amrap

10 Russian KB swings
200m run
10 pushups

KB WOD 144
3 rounds:
9 dual KB situps
7 dual KB push press
5 dual KB bent over row

KB WOD 145
2 rounds:
30 situps
20 Russian KB twists
10 seated KB presses
400m run

KB WOD 146
5-5-5-5-5
dual kb deadlift (bodyweight)
Hold as many KBs as necessary

KB WOD 147

10 rounds:

3 clean & press

6 pushups

9 air squats

KB WOD 148

6 rounds:

4 KB deadlift

3 KB cleans from the ground

2 KB squat cleans

1 KB thruster

KB WOD 149

20 minute amrap

5 KB deadlift

10 KB American wing

15 KB Russian swing

200m run

KB WOD 150

10 rounds:

7 American swings

5 burpees

KB WOD 151

5 rounds:

21 KB American swings

250m run

12 Ring Dips

KB WOD 152

4 rounds:

50 KB American swings

40 KB Russian twists

30 KB wall ball

KB WOD 153

5 rounds:

15 KB American swings

5 burpees

KB WOD 154

2 rounds:

1 TGU

150m run

2 TGU

150m run

3 TGU

150m run

2 TGU

150m run
1 TGU

KB WOD 155
21-15-9
KB thrusters
pullups

KB WOD 156
2 rounds:
7-5-3
KB deadlift
KB press
KB thruster
400m run

KB WOD 157
400m run
10 dual KB squat cleans
30 burpees
600m run
20 dual KB squat cleans
20 burpees
800m run
30 dual KB squat cleans
10 burpees

KB WOD 158
4 rounds:
30 KB clean and Press

KB WOD 159
5 Deadlift
10 Swing
200m run

KB WOD 160
21-15-9
push-ups
thrusters
sit-ups
200m run

KB WOD 161
2 rounds:
800m run
21 KB snatch
15 KB American swings
9 TGUs
800m run

KB WOD 162

9 minute amrap

7 dual KB cleans from the swing

5 push ups

3 knee to elbows

KB WOD 163

3 rounds:

30 box jump

30 American swing

400m run

KB WOD 164

4 rounds:

5 KB cleans to lunge

10 American swings

400m run

KB WOD 165

4 rounds:

400m run

21 American swings

12 pullups

KB WOD 166
50-30-20
clean and press (each arm)
ab mat situps
Russian swings

KB WOD 167
3 rounds:
21 pull ups
15 dual KB swing to clean and press
400m run

KB WOD 168
2 rounds:
50-30-20
1 arm Russian swing
double unders

KB WOD 169
1000m row
50 snatches

800m run
50 American wwings

KB WOD 170
7 rounds:
7 dual KB deadlifts
7 burpees
7 pullups

KB WOD 171
45 KB snatch
400m run
35 KB snatch
400m run
25 KB snatch
400m run
reps are total, divide for each arm

KB WOD 172
15 minute amrap
5 dual KB clean
5 dual KB push press
5 dual KB front squat

KB WOD 173

21-15-9
American swings
pushups
Russian twist

KB WOD 174

100 American Swings
50 Sit-ups
50 American Swings
100 Sit-ups

KB WOD 175

2 rounds:
50 Russian swings
40 jump squats
30 Russian twists
20 KB situps
10 pushups

KB WOD 176

3 rounds:
800m run

12 KB push press
24 American swings
800m run

KB WOD 177

3 rounds:

400m row

30 Russian swings

10 pushups

KB WOD 178

3 rounds:

300m row

30 Russian swings

10 burpees

KB WOD 179

3 rounds:

200m row

30 Russian swings

10 pushups

KB WOD 180

15 minute amrap

3 snatch

5 overhead squat
7 push press

KB WOD 181
2 rounds:
50 Russian swings
800m run
50 Russian swings
500m row
50 Russian swings

KB WOD 182
2 rounds:
50 push press
50 American swings
100ft KB lunge
35 push press
35 American swings
100ft KB lunge
20 push press
20 American swings
100ft KB lunge
400m KB farmers walk

KB WOD 183

400m run

50 Russian swings

800m run

35 Russian swings

800m run

20 Russian swings

400m run

KB WOD 184

REPS 20-16-12-8-4

KB front squat

KB snatch

burpees

KB WOD 185

50-40-30

Russian swing

pushups

squats

KB WOD 186

4 rounds:

25 dual KB clean and press

300m row

KB WOD 187

For time:

800m run

20 KB deadlifts

20 pushups

20 KB power swings

800m run

KB WOD 188

4 rounds:

11 burpees

21 Dual KB cleans

jump rope – 100 skips

11 American swings

11 situps

800m run

KB WOD 189

1000m row

21-15-9

Dual KB Snatch

burpees

KB WOD 190

30-20-10

dual KB press

dual KB clean

dual KB lunge

25 KB walking lunges

25 KB snatch

800m run

25 KB walking lunges

25 KB snatch

KB WOD 191

3 rounds:

35 American swings

100m power skip

15 pushups

KB WOD 192

3 rounds:

15 KB clean and press

200m run

21 knee to elbow

KB WOD 193

7 rounds:
7 KB deadlifts
7 Russian swings
7 pullups

KB WOD 194

15 burpees
35 American swings
800m farmers walk
15 burpees
35 American swings

KB WOD 195

5 rounds:
21 American swings
15 squats
9 pushups

KB WOD 196

15 minute amrap
12 KB cleans
200m run
12 KB snatch to overhead squat

KB WOD 197

2 rounds:

400m run

25 American swings

25 ring dips

25 walking lunge

25 ring dips

25 American swings

400m run

KB WOD 198

2 rounds:

800m run

44 American Swing

22 Russian Swing

11 Burpees

800m run

KB WOD 199

2 rounds:

3 rounds

400m run

21 American Swings

12 Pullups

KB WOD 200

15 minute amrap
12 dual KB deadlift
9 dual KB cleans
6 dual KB front Squat
3 dual KB push press

KB WOD 201

box jump
21,18,15,12,9,6
American swings
6,9,12,15,18,21

KB WOD 202

3 rounds:
20 Russian swings
5 burpees
10 clean and press
20 situps
400m sprint

KB WOD 203

4 rounds:
400m run

15 American swings
10 snatch to overhead squat

KB WOD 204
15 minute amrap
15 Russian swings
10 dual KB front squat

KB WOD 205
5 rounds
15 box jumps
10 single arm swings (each arm)
15 pushups
10 KB push press (each arm)

Bonus WODs

On the following pages you will find 20 assorted bonus WODs, these include Olympic, hybrid and bodyweight exercises.

BONUS WOD 1

Time trial:

Run 10km

BONUS WOD 2

Intervals:

Rest 2 minutes between intervals

Row 6x500m

BONUS WOD 3

5 rounds:

Rest as needed between rounds

Back squat 5-5-3-3-1x

BONUS WOD 4

Intervals:

Row 4x1200m

Rest 2 minutes between intervals

BONUS WOD 5

5 rounds for total reps:

45 seconds Box jumps (18 inch)

15 seconds rest

45 seconds Box jumps (24 inch)

15 seconds rest

45 seconds Box jumps (30 inch)
90 seconds rest

BONUS WOD 6

Every minute on the minute for 12 minutes:

1x Deadlift

3x Burpees

5x KB swings

BONUS WOD 7

Every minute on the minute for max rounds:

From the rack start with 1x jerk (50% 1RM)

Add 5 lbs each successive minute, continue until failure

BONUS WOD 8

Every minute on the minute for max rounds:

3x Back squat

5x Strict pull-ups

sprint 40 yards

Each minute thereafter add 1 rep to your squat, continue until failure

BONUS WOD 9

Every minute on the minute for 15 minutes:

3x Power clean

5x Box jumps (30 inch)

10x Push-ups

BONUS WOD 10

Every minute on the minute for max rounds:

5x Box jump (20 inch)

7x Sumo Deadlift high pull

9x Push press

BONUS WOD 11

AMRAP in 12 minutes:
5x Ground to overhead
10x Floor wipers
15x Lateral hops over BB

BONUS WOD 12

6 rounds:
5x Hang power clean
30 yard sprint
Bear crawl back to start

BONUS WOD 13

AMRAP in 15 minutes:
3x Thruster
6x Box jump
9x KB swings

BONUS WOD 14

For time:
Run 1000m
100x Push-ups
10x Snatch

BONUS WOD 15

5 rounds:

8x KB clean & jerk

8x Burpees

8x Strict pull-ups

BONUS WOD 16

3 rounds:

20x Double-unders

20x Floor wipers

20x Back extensions

20x MB twists

20x Knees-to-elbows

20x Decline sit-ups

BONUS WOD 17

3 rounds:

Run 400m

40x Walking lunge steps

30x Sit ups

20x Push ups

10x Burpees

BONUS WOD 18

3 rounds each:

3x Bench press

10x Plyo push-ups

5x Back squat

6x Box jumps (24 inch)

BONUS WOD 19

For time:

25x Back squat

50x Box jump (24 inch)

75x Wall ball

100x Squats

BONUS WOD 20

3 rounds:
15x Burpees
20x Sit-ups
45x Push-ups
60x Squats
Run 400m

Conclusion

I hope you have found this book useful, as you can now see incorporating kettlebells in your daily workouts have a plethora of benefits, I highly recommend you put down the dumbbells for a while and implement some kettlebell based training in your regime.

By following these workouts on a regular basis you'll develop not only a strong, flexible, functionally fit body that'll be ready to tackle any situation life throws at it but also an unbreakable mindset and confidence to match.

I hope you enjoyed reading this book as much as I enjoyed writing it.

P.S

34183196R00063

Printed in Great Britain
by Amazon